THE HCG METABOLISM TREATMENT

OVER 30 KILOS IN WEIGHT LOSS? – I HAVE DONE IT, AND YOU CAN DO IT AS WELL!

FRANK SCHMIDT

Copyright © Frank Schmidt
All Rights Reserved.

ISBN 978-1-63957-059-1

This book has been published with all efforts taken to make the material error-free after the consent of the author. However, the author and the publisher do not assume and hereby disclaim any liability to any party for any loss, damage, or disruption caused by errors or omissions, whether such errors or omissions result from negligence, accident, or any other cause.

While every effort has been made to avoid any mistake or omission, this publication is being sold on the condition and understanding that neither the author nor the publishers or printers would be liable in any manner to any person by reason of any mistake or omission in this publication or for any action taken or omitted to be taken or advice rendered or accepted on the basis of this work. For any defect in printing or binding the publishers will be liable only to replace the defective copy by another copy of this work then available.

Contents

Foreword — v

1. What Does Hcg Mean And What Is A Hcg-diet? — 1
2. The Four Phases Of The Hcg-metabolic Cure — 5
3. Hcg Intestinal Cleansing And Hcg-metabolic Cure — 6
4. Active Components Used — 9
5. Let's Go! — 16
6. The Procedure — 28
7. Epilogue And Sources — 30
8. Bibliography — 32

Disclaimer — 37

Foreword

Dear readers,

My book »The hCG Bowel Cleansing« is by now available at bookshops and I was astonished by how many people had already purchased the printed or digital edition, since I am neither a diet guru nor a doctor, but have only written down my own dieting experiences.

In large part, this is certainly also due to my pride in my accomplishment. For anyone, who, like myself, had been struggling with overweight for decades, it is a great accomplishment to make such significant progress of getting more than 30 kilos closer to your ideal weight in a relatively short period of time.

Another reason why I started writing down my experiences was that I wanted to encourage those people who suffer from overweight. There are ways to permanently lose weight and maintain the new one. Maybe it is easier for you to believe this coming from a person affected, than from some nutritionist, whose dieting experience is limited to losing two kilos after Christmas?

What's great about this whole story is: it continues. Of course, I have adjusted my eating habits during the time of my weight reduction. Nevertheless: I basically still eat everything I like: this sometimes may include Italian salami as much as a piece of chocolate every now and again. There is no pressure to diet in my life. However, during the time I did the hCG metabolism treatment my attitude towards food has changed as well. Above all, I noticed that today I am more conscious of what I eat. The result: just yesterday I noticed that my pants, which two months ago fight rather tightly, now began to slip even with a belt on.

FOREWORD

If you suffer from overweight, I just want to tell you: I believe from the bottom of my heart that with time you are able to reach a healthy weight. I wish you great success in reaching your goal and I hope my book will support you in the process.

Good luck with your weight loss,

Your Frank Schmidt

PPS: Even though this book is an experience report, I am aware that there may be some readers who would like to better understand my experiences themselves. Please do so only after consulting the practitioner of your trust. I am not a practitioner and no nutritionist, and even though the methods I used were successful for me, I cannot evaluate how they will affect your body!

ONE
WHAT DOES HCG MEAN AND WHAT IS A HCG-DIET?

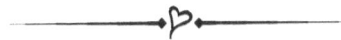

In the midst of the 20th century, an English doctor named Albert Theodore William Simeons (1902-1970) made an interesting discovery. After he had finished his studies at the University of Heidelberg »Summa cum Laude« and worked in a large hospital near Dresden, he deepened his studies in the field of tropical diseases, first worked in Africa for two years and finally moved to India in 1931, where he stayed for 18 years.

Dr. Simeons discovered a treatment for Malaria, which he received honour for from the Queen. After the Indian Independence, Dr. Simeons founded his own medial practice in Bombay, until he moved on to Rome with his family in 1949, where he worked on healing psychosomatic illnesses in the » Salvator Mundi International Hospital« until his death in 1970.

Besides these topics, there was another central research topic in the life of the doctor. He spent some three decades of his life searching for the causes of obesity and finally found what he had been looking for through the evaluation of data of an Indian pregnant woman.

Simeons realized that these hard working women, who often carried out hard labour on the fields for the whole day and did not eat a lot themselves, gave birth to healthy children of normal weight. The women hardly felt hungry and their offsprings were not affected.

Indeed, Dr. Simeons could prove that the notion that a pregnant woman had to eat for two was completely wrong. In contrast, it is absolutely sufficient for the mother to eat normally (and healthy). This provides her the chance to even reduce her own bodyweight during pregnancy, without harming the baby at all.

Several years of research allowed Dr. Simeons to prove that the effect was clearly caused by an endogenous substance called hCG (humanChorionic Gonadotropin). hCGis a glycoprotein. It is produced in the placenta during pregnancy in order to ensure the nutrition of the foetus.

Dr. Simeons subsequently tried to find out whether the consumption of hCG may also lead to a loss of weight in non-pregnant people, and gave hCG to obese boys. In all cases, these procedures lead to success.

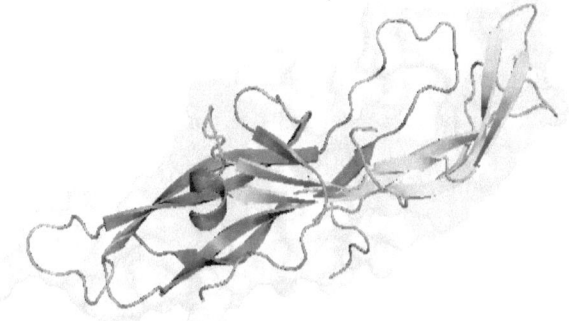

It was remarkable, that only adipose fat so the fat at the problem zones was released, but not the fat that protects organs and hinges or that corresponds to the normal fat reserves of the organism.

In his clinic, Dr. Simeons developed his diet further and combined hCG-giving (at the time in form of injections, today drops, globules or other forms are standard) with a specific 500 calories diet.

This is achieved because hCG affects the hypothalamus of the human. This is the controlling unit for our metabolism. There is also defined, which weight is "normal" for the human. This point is called, "Setpoint". The body does everything it can, to try and hold this weight.

If the weight is adjusted in a normal diet, but the Setpoint stays the same (the body only adjusts it over a long period of time), the body tries to reach that point again.

Weight gain is inevitable.

Since hCG adjusts the Setpoint together with the weight reduction, a new weight gain is prevented (except if you overdraw extremely), so the body tries to hold this lower Setpoint.

The hCG metabolism culture, as I implemented it, consists of 3 basic components, that optimally work together.

- Adjustment of the Setpoint through hCG
- Adjustment of weight through change in diet
- Optimization of physical health and supply of required vitamins, to cover the increased demand through the increased metabolism (fat burning)

In the following text, I will name concrete products. Not because I think of them as the only ones possible to get the same results as I did, but because these are experience reports and I want to be as transparent as possible. I took hCG in my two own diets in different forms, as drops and also in form of salt. The vitamins which I took are from the company Lifeplus. I chose this provider because of the high quality of their products and because of recommendations.

A lot of which I have lost.

TWO

The four phases of the hCG-Metabolic Cure

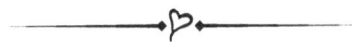

The hCG-Metabolic Cure, depending on the users, can be divided into two to four different phases. In essence, though, the meaning is the same; it is handled more on the question of what one would like summarized. There I have divided the diet into 4 phases, each with their different themes. This has also the advantage in that through this process everyone who wishes to begin an hCG-Intestinal cleansing has a clear entry point.

THREE
HCG Intestinal Cleansing and HCG-Metabolic Cure

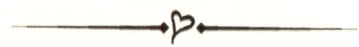

How does an hCG-Colon Cleanse stand in relation to the hCG-Metabolic Cure?

I myself have had my first diet round with the hCG-Metabolic Cure and within the first three weeks (21 days of the diet phases) have lost a dozen kilograms. Per day, that's more than half a kilo-which I have found to be remarkable. So, to me this is reason enough to immediately begin the hCG- Metabolic Cure. I was successful with it and have found nothing but conclusive results. Because of this, I have written this book on the topic of the hCG-Metabolic Cure

By undertaking the hCG-Metabolic Cure, I have read and learned much about our intestines. Yes, I understand that it is a body part that few people would like to give thought to. Nevertheless, I have done it and have read Julia Ende's book

»Darm mit Charme«, which has led me to fall in love with this unloved „Hose".

I have written in my first book „ The HCG Gut Cleansing: Your basis for double success in your metabolism cure. - Why a metabolism cure after intestinal cleansing is much more successful. ":

My first foray into the theme of Intestinal Cleansing was very easy. I imagined how it would most likely be if I tried to fertilize my lawn with the world's best fertilizer- but in winter, when the lawn would be buried under 20 centimeters of snow. Only a fraction of the fertilizer would be able to cut through the snow and reach the lawn. The majority of it would carried carry away by melted snow.

It is the same with our intestines if toxins begin to overlay it, old fecal stones begin to accumulate in the bowel pockets, which can allow for bacteria and fungi to overrun the bowels. Even with the best nutritional diet, full doses of vitamins and supplements can be transformed in this type of atmosphere into putrid mud, which hinders the body's processing of them.

If I only – staying on my image of a lawn – had some patience, I would have proceeded as follows: I would first let the law have some exposure, or better yet wait, until the snow had melted away into the grass. Then, I would only need a fraction of the world's best fertilizer, and it would still have more success in fertilizing my lawn than if I had tried when there was 20 centimeters of snow.

This was my exact strategy before I began my second take on changing my metabolic rate. I would first make my intestinal system as receptive.

I highly recommend you start your hCG-Intestinal Cleansing now.

In the second pass of my diet, I lost weight quicker and easier than when I used the classic hCG-metabolism-culture. Or you could start with the hCG-colon-cleanse first and then the first phase with the hCG-metabolism-culture. Both are possible. All you need to know, you will find in said book.

Here I only describe the classical hCG-metabolism-culture, like I used it myself first.

FOUR
Active Components Used

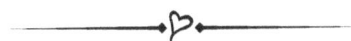

The following product, of course, is not the only ones possible. I'd rather like to be transparent in the scope of my documentation and to show concretely what helped me. This seems especially important to me because I'm aware of the bad quality that many suppliers in the supplement industry provide. For this reason (and because of recommendation of a colleague), I decided to use products of LifePlus and didn't regret this. It's the result that counts, after all.

Vitamin and Mineral Supply

The basis for diet success is a basic vitamin and mineral supply. The body needs them to do its work optimally. The better our cells work, the more calories they burn. Especially during a diet, where we consume even less food, it's important to provide additional vitamins. For this, I took 1 tablet of LifePlus TVM Plus in the morning, one on midday and one in the evening.

Summary:

3x2 tablets a day (before the meals respectively), daily during the whole diet (all 4 phases)

Cell Protection and Back-Formation of Skin

I admit that I could use the topic of cell protection very much and took the product LifePlus Proanthenols 100 mainly because of a colleague that recommended the treatment. For this reason, I started to read different books about the topic myself. There I found documented positive impacts on vessels, blood circuit, allergies, eyes, skin, blood values, respiration ducts, and mood.

This is undoubtedly a wide range of positive effects. What I am particularly impressed about and can fully support from own experience also, are the positive effects on skin and mood. The others are also given, but since I had no such impairments before cure, I can't leave a statement for that.

What I noticed very well (I take Life Plus Proanthenols 100 even after the diet continued) is, that my skin regressed very well. Of course, that did not work from one day to the other, but through the positive effect on the collagen in the skin, it increased skin elasticity and the period in which I had to fight with hanging flaps of skin was extremely short. Compared to a diet without Proanthenols 100 I saved myself a larger, costly operation and, therefore, I thank my colleague sincerely that he did not let loose.

From a friend who also took the same substance, I have been told that she found a very positive effect on cellulite and stretch marks. She told me that she finally goes back into the pool without inhibitions. Also: a great success, I think.

The second positive impact of Proanthenols in my diet was its mood-lifting effect. What I've always really hated with diets was the fact that I was always somehow being depressed. It was almost as if my subconscious mourns after every single kilo. A stupid situation! This time - probably by taking Proanthenols–I felt so splendidly that even my friends noticed.

Summary:

3x1 compact Proanthenols 100 (morning / noon / evening) daily for all diet phases (1-4)

Essential fatty acids

A wonderful quote about Omega 3 I initially found in the book "I had discovered a fat bag" by Christoph Bisel. It originally came from Prof. Hamm and Dirk Neuberger[2]:

»Overweight people, however, should by no means go without the supporting effect of EPA/DHA during the weight reduction. Fish consumption or omega-3 fatty acids improve the increased risk of overweight patients for cardiovascular diseases as they lower blood lipid levels and help normalize the blood glucose-insulin metabolism. (...) Especially in regards to this risk constellation, the inclusion of meals containing omega-3 fatty acids reinforces the effect of weight reduction beyond the already expected extent of your weight loss.« Furthermore, they write: *»And for those who still want to cut down on calories even more strictly, can always resort to capsules, which contain the healthy fatty acids in concentrated form. «*

Through the daily intake of two capsules of LifePlus OmeGold I have, myself noticed an increase in cognitive performance and the absence of energy loss during the day, which otherwise often occurs during diets. For me OmeGold was my insurance - so to speak, in order to be able to go on living normally and be able to successfully fulfill my daily duties (and work) during my diet.

Summary:

2 capsules LifePlus Omegold daily in the morning (in all diet phases)

Detoxification

Do you know the typical diet face? Dark circles around the eyes, a weary look ... anyone who has done an intense diet over a longer period of time exactly knows this face from the mirror. Even the magic of make-up for the ladies reaches its limits during such times. On top of that, there is also crankiness, lack of motivation and possibly even joint pain? You remember?

Taking a closer look, you can see that these are symptoms of intoxication. We all take in toxins from our surrounding world each day. This can happen by inhaling air, eating food or through our skin. Our body fights this by storing these substances in our fat cells and thereby gets rid of them because it can't manage to dispose of all of them any other way.

When we dissolve fat cells in the course of a diet, this has the negative side effect of releasing these toxins, and because in many people these substances are enclosed in their fat cells, their level of toxins in the blood goes up and leads to cells being attacked.

By taking LifePlus MSM, I have put a compound against this to use. MSM stands for Methylsulfonylmethane. Wikipedia.de states the following:

Methylsulfonylmethane is found in many animal and vegetable organisms and is also a part of human nutrition. High concentrations are found in cow's milk (3.3 ppm) and in coffee (1.6 ppm)

In his book »The BMI-Coach Metabolism Treatment«[1]Christoph Bisel writes the following in regard to this substance:

Since I started my diet, I started taking MSM as well. Experts say that it makes sense to take MSM at least for six months in addition to actual diet, because it´s purpose is eliminating poisons that were previously stored in fat and are being released during the diet. In the USA, MSM is being used for a long time in naturopathic practices as part of a mild strategy against inflammation, pain, and other ailments. In the context of metabolism cure, MSM is taken to prevent the usual negative consequences of diets, resulting from the re-deposition of the released toxins. Otherwise, there is a risk that the relevant pollutants can be stored in organ tissue, fat, brain and bone marrow. This leads in many cases to the fact that people who make conventional diets are pale, have dark circles around the eyes, have joint pains and feel bad in general.

One particularly nice side effect of the intake of MSM during this time is for me the fact that the gingivitis, which was normally present in the area of my prosthesis, didn´t happen since then.

In fact, I continued using MSM after my last diet, which was even several months ago. In my opinion, this substance in any case belongs to every home remedy kit, due to it´s positive effects associated with inflammation.

I started the daily intake with three tablets a day (1 tablet in the morning, noon, and evening) and then, depending on diet phase, I moved on to six and finally to nine tablets a day. I continued doing this throughout the whole diet and only after I gradually reduced it again. The first three months I continued to take 3x2 tablets and then 3x 1 tablets.

Summary:

Daily intake: 3 x 1 tablet LifePlus MSM a day (morning, noon, evening)

1st week of the diet phase: 3 x 2 tablets LifePlus MSM a day (morning, noon, evening)

Rest of the diet: 3 x 3 tablets LifePlus MSM a day (morning, noon, evening)

My secret ingredient: Magnesium

I´ve encountered magnesium to support my diet by my reading during the diet. In fact, statistics show that a large proportion of people in our culture are suffering a massive magnesium deficiency. This is particularly significant because magnesium is mainly important for the way we deal with external influences, from stress to attacks of diseases. Stress or anger consumes about 50 mg of magnesium and sodas quasi-rinse it from the body.

Let us make no mistake. Dieting is stressful for the body, but also for "the soul," regardless the method we use.

Magnesium deficiency manifests itself in apathy, insomnia, sleeping problems, cramps in the legs, fatigue. Some doctors are also convinced that the continuously increasing number of burnout cases has a reason in a long-lasting, solid magnesium deficiency of the patient concerned. One of my acquaintance doctor, who treats those affected, said to me once: "Not everyone who suffers from magnesium deficiency, is also suffering from burnout. But the number of people with burnout, which I treated so far and which did not suffer from magnesium deficiency, I can count on the fingers of one hand. "

This is certainly no clinical study, but it should make us think.

In the context of a weight reduction, another aspect about magnesium is important to notice. It's a leading part of fat reduction. Each single cell needs magnesium to work properly. If the cell is undersupplied, it cuts back its functions and therefore also the burning of calories.

For this reason, I took 3 tablets of LifePlusCalMag Plus daily in my diet (and also continued). Those tablets also contain other important elements such as alfalfa, phosphorus, zinc, copper, manganese, and so on.

Summary:

3x2 tablets a day (one before each meal) while sticking to the diet (all 4 phases)

FIVE

LET'S GO!

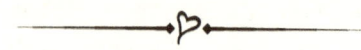

As described earlier, the hCG-metaboliccure is made from three elements: the setting of the set point, a weight reduction and the intake of necessary vital substances. Actually this combination is central. One could think that it's already enough to reduce the weight by reducing calories and to make sure by taking hCG, that the setpoint is established at a low level. In fact, there are basic approaches which propagate exactly that. But this approach would mean to shoot our own efforts into the foot.

The success of the metabolic cure is based to a certain degree in activating the metabolism and burning more calories by that. This metabolism happens in our body cells and means a substantial excess work. Now there is the problem, that most of our diseases of civilization were proven to root in malnutrition of many cells with important substances and vitamins, magnesium and other minerals.

Who tries to accelerate the metabolism by a metabolic cure and does not consider that the cell also needs more vital substances, robs the cells by their ability to burn calories at full capacity. At the same time, the malnutrition of the cell (which might already have existed before) for a certain time means an increased potential of damage.

The hCG-metabolic cure is made up by 4 stages. Those absolutely must be adhered to in time and order to have the full success and to make sure that the setpoint and other physical sentiments as the feeling of satiety are adjusted to the situation.

Stage 1: Days of loading

The days of loading don't really look like a diet. Two days of full and feudal eating in combination with three doses of hCG. This really sounds exotic.

But basically this approach has two important reasons and is crucial for the success in this diet:

A multitude of diets runs out of energy after a few days because the body goes into Standby-Mode to save energy. But especially doing a diet based in the increase of the metabolism, this is counterproductive. Those two days of gluttony are signaling to the body that there is sufficient food supply available and he doesn't have to »switch« modes.

The psychological effect of the days of loading is at least equal in its importance in this diet. In fact, the hCG decreases the sensation of hunger, once a sufficient level is reached. This effect is supported by the sensation of repleteness. I at least experienced it like a relief when after two days of gluttony finally the diet stage started and I could give my body some rest.

Take care that you don't eat too late even on the loading days. A too ample gut prevents from sleeping and getting enough sleep is an important factor for the success of any diet.

The vital substances during the loading days:

During my two loading days I used the following nutrients to support my diet:

- 3 times a day one unit hCG Drops

Different providers offer these as drops, salt or globules. Select the quantities based on the manufacturer's specifications.

- 3 times daily 2 tablets of Lifeplus TVM Plus
- 3 times daily 1 tablet of Lifeplus Proanthenols 100
- 2 capsules Lifeplus OmeGold in the morning
- 3 times daily 1 tablet of Lifeplus MSM Plus
- 3 times daily 2 tablets Lifeplus CalMag

Phase 2: Diet Phase:

Now that you feasted two days, the actual diet starts. In fact, here we talk about a calorie count of 500 to 700 calories a day. This is an amount that might give an experienced counter of calories quite a headache. "How can you only live by those few calories then? As I will starve to death before reaching my ideal weight," I was thinking, as I told my friend of the metabolism cure.

In fact, I couldn't be more wrong. In all the time of my diet, I never felt hungry on any single day. The reason lies in a "side effect" of hCG, which will greatly reduce the feeling of hunger or shut it completely off. Apart from this, another aim of the whole diet is to suggest to the body that one cannot "live off the calories consumed," just that the body has the incentive of burning all the stored fuel (let's call it shorter: fats)

The diet phase - as well as the next two phases - takes at least 21 days. This is because the experience taught us that the body needs that time for saving new programs. This is of central importance for setting up the new setpoints. It is possible to stretch each of the phases to more than 21 days, which basically makes sense to perform multiple metabolic cures successive at larger "projects". Like this, you give the body the opportunity to adapt well to the new realities. In particular the skin has the opportunity to

regress gradually.

Nutritional daily schedule

The 500-700 calories are distributed as follows:
Time
Ingestion
Daytime
Min. 2 Lt. of Water
For breakfast
1-2 Cups of unsweetened coffee or tea without milk
For brunch
1 fruit
For lunch
120-130g proteins and vegetables
For the afternoon
1 fruit
For dinner
120-130g proteins and vegetables
In the evening

1 cup of unsweetened coffee or tea

1 glass of water with fresh squeezed lemon juice (unsweetened)

If possible, avoid any foods you didn't cook by yourself. Some additives, such as sugars, aspartame, and various others as well as glutamine may affect the success of our diet considerably.

To keep your metabolism busy overnight, I (unsweetened, of course) drink the juice of a freshly squeezed lemon in a glass of water late in the evening. Who, therefore, cannot sleep, should omit it.

Food Table

Suitable proteins (always pay attention to the number of calories!)

- Beef (lean)
- Veal (lean)
- Ostrich meat (lean)
- Lean poultry meat
- White, low-fat fish (cod, halibut, gilthead, pike, sole, anglerfish)
- Seafood and shellfish
- Eggs
- Cottage cheese, curd cheese and yoghurt (lean)
- Tofu

Unsuitable proteins

- Pork
- Sausage
- Ham

- Goose
- Duck
- Lamb
- Oily fish (herring, salmon, eel, mackerel, and all smoked fish or fish pickled in oil)
- Full-fat dairy products
- Cheese (except cottage cheese)

Suitable vegetables and salads

- Aubergine (eggplant)
- Lettuces
- Cauliflower
- Chicory
- Chinese cabbage
- Fennel
- Spring onions
- Green beans
- Kale
- Leek
- Kohlrabi
- Pak choi
- Peppers
- Parsley root
- Mushrooms
- Radishes
- Brussels sprouts
- Red Cabbage
- Cucumbers
- Celery
- Asparagus
- Spinach
- Tomatoes (no cocktail tomatoes)

- White cabbage
- Savoy cabbage
- Zucchini (courgette)

- Onions

Unsuitable vegetables and salads

- Avocados
- Beans
- Peas
- Carrots
- Potatoes
- Lentils
- Corn

Suitable fruits

- Apples (sour)
- Blueberries
- Strawberries
- Grapefruit (pomelo)
- Oranges
- Papaya
- Rhubarb
- Red currants

Unsuitable fruits

- Pineapple !
- Apricots
- Bananas

- Pears
- Cherries
- Peaches
- Grapes
- All kinds of dried fruits

Suitable drinks

- Water (non-carbonated, without flavoring enhancers and sweeteners)
- Coffee (max. 1x daily, if possible without milk)
- Black tea
- Green tea
- Mate tea
- Pu-erh tea
- Herbal teas

Unsuitable beverage

- Alcohol
- Non-alcoholic beer
- Energy drinks (not even the "calorie-free")
- Sodas
- Milk
- Fruit juices
- Smoothies

Suitable spices

- Aceto Balsamico
- Apple Cider Vinegar
- Curry

- Garam Masala
- Vegetable broth (fat-free)
- Ginger
- Herbs (fresh or dried)
- Turmeric
- Horseradish (fresh or from a glass, without sugar and cream)
- Paprika
- Pepper
- Saffron
- Salt (use sea salt or Himalayan salt)
- Sambal Oelek (without sugar)
- Mustard (without added sugar)
- Soy sauce (limited)
- Stevia
- Tabasco
- Tomato paste (without added sugar)
- Wasabi
- Cinnamon
- Lemon juice

Unsuitable spices

- Artificial Sweeteners
- Glutamate
- Sodium chloride
- Flavor enhancers
- Sauces and condiments (often contain preservatives, sugars or glutamate).

Spicy flavoring stimulates the metabolism and is, therefore, positive. Spicy should not be confused with salty.

The vital substances in the diet phase

The intake of hCG has been continued from the loading days. Furthermore, a dose has been taken three times daily. Especially in this phase the goal is to adjust the set points and this is made possible by taking the hCG.

During my two loading days I have used the following products to support my diet:

- 3 x daily one unit of hCG drops

Different providers offer these as drops, salt or globules. Select the quantities based on the manufacturer's specifications.

- 3 x daily 2 tablets LifePlus TVM Plus
- 3 x daily 1 tablet Lifeplus Proanthenols 100
- 2 capsules Lifeplus OmeGold in the mornings
- 3 x daily 2 tablets Lifeplus MSM Plus in the first week, then 3 tablets 3 times a day.
- 3 x daily 2 tablets Lifeplus CalMag Plus

Phase 3: Stabilization Phase

The stabilization phase was for me the greatest challenge. On the one hand, the intake of HCG has been discontinued in order to anchor the Setpoint at the low level, which didn't lead directly to hunger, but meant a certain conversion of the body at the end of the diet phase. On the other hand, I found that after the diet phase in which I had pulled myself together, there was "a little air out of the balloon." It took an enormous amount of energy to motivate me to endure this phase.

In the stabilization phase, it is important that the body adapts to the new weight and that another Setpoint is anchored. At this stage, I have increased my calorie intake gradually again until 1000, and finally to about 1400 kcal.

Apart from carbohydrates and ready meals with additives everything is permitted (which falls within the calorie range).

The stabilization phase should also be carried out for three weeks.

The Steak Day

During the stabilization phase, there will be fluctuations of approximately one kilo. This is normal and depends, for example, on bowel movements and other processes in your body. If you are gaining more than 1 kilo, it is worthwhile to insert a Steak day.

Additionally, you must only eat a small steak or if you want, Beefsteak-Tartar in the afternoon and evening. Coming to spices, you should avoid too much salt and preferably flavor more with fresh herbs, pepper or chili. Seasoning with glutamate and similar additives is taboo during the whole diet.

After Steak day, the body usually returns to your newly programmed weight.

The vital substances during the stabilization phase

Attention, important: no longer take hCG!

- 3 times daily 2 pills Lifeplus TVM Plus
- 3 x 1 pills daily Lifeplus Proanthenols 100
- 2 capsules Lifeplus OmeGold morning
- 3 x daily 3 pills Lifeplus MSM Plus
- 3 times daily 2 pills Lifeplus CalMag Plus

Phase 4: Test phase

The Test phase is the natural continuation of the stabilization period. The aim of test phase is that you start to test different foods and to see how your body reacts to them. Usually, again 3 weeks are scheduled for that.

Each body is different and other foods are better for it (or not). Right now, it's important for you to find out which foods you should keep an eye on. It is a fact that some people struggle with overweight, because of incompatibility. That's why it makes a lot of sense to find out, if you have any and if so, to avoid these kinds of products.

The vital substances during the testing phase

The vital substances of the stabilization phase will still be taken to the same extent:

- 3 x daily 2 pills LifePlus TVM Plus
- 3 x daily 1 pill LifePlus Proanthenols 100
- 2 capsules LifePlus Omegold in the Morning
- 3 x daily 3 pills Lifeplus MSM Plus
- 3 x daily 2 pills LifePlus CalMag Plus

SIX

THE PROCEDURE

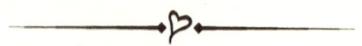

Let me shortly outline the two options of the diet, on the one hand, the version with the hCG-bowel-cleanse, that I described in my first book, and, on the other hand, the »pure« hCG-metabolic-cure, that I successfully conducted during my first round:

The hCG-metabolic-cure procedure

If you implement the hCG-metabolic-cure in combination with a hCG-bowel-cleanse, this has proven to be good for me:

30 days hCG-bowel-cleanse (like I described in my 1st book)

21 days phase 3 (stabilizing phase) of the hCG- metabolic-cure

21 days phase 4 (testing phase) der hCG- metabolic-cure

If you didn't lose enough weight with this, let your body rest for at least 3 – 4 Weeks (still take your vital substances) and afterwards begin with a normal hCG-metabolic-cure.

The »normal« procedure

The hCG-metabolic-cure without the hCG-bowel-cleanse is quasi the standard procedure, as described by different authors and has also been successfully implemented by me. With that, I lost 12 kilo in 3 weeks. Not bad, isn't it?

The Procedure is:

2 days phase 1: load-days

21 days phase 2: diet-days (there is a possibility to do this even longer, but you have much better and more sustainable success if you stay with 21 days and perform a new hCG-metabolic-cure afterwards, if needed.)

21 days phase 3: stabilizing phase

21 days phase 4: testing phase

If needed, the entire process can be repeated. I recommend though having at least a 3-4 week break between regiments. This has advantages in that it allows for a phase of „normal living" in which your body can refill and recharge, and it also gives your body more time to switch to a new environment/situation. In particular, it is also advisable so that your skin can better rebuild itself.

SEVEN

Epilogue and Sources

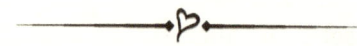

I sincerely hope that this book has answered many questions and has raised your level of motivation and activity to prevent over weightiness.

In parallel with this epilogue, I have begun work on a new book. It should better explain and enlighten those about the time after one completes an hCG-Metabolic Cure. But even I cannot give an exact date as to when the book will be available. In any case, I would very glad to count you among my readers.

As with the previous book, I am also excited to hear any feedback you may have, because I consider you also „my "source for Lifeplus Products (I myself am only a consumer, offering nothing to it).

You can reach me by mail under **hcgdarm@gmail.com**.

I will always try to answer as soon as possible. Depending on the number of incoming mails though, I may need a few days to respond.

I recently have come across a book by a Dan Hill called "How to accelerate your metabolism? A healthy and sustainable way to loose additional weight":

I found it to be very exciting to see what further possibilities are available to optimize the cure, and I would without a doubt try them when I am ready to lose my next few kilos.

EIGHT

BIBLIOGRAPHY

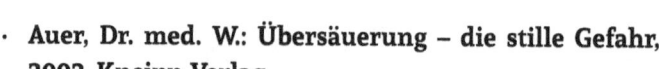

- Auer, Dr. med. W.: Übersäuerung – die stille Gefahr, 2002, Kneipp-Verlag
- Arndt, U.: Spirulina, Chlorella, AFA-Algen: Lichtvolle Power-Nahrung für Körper und Geist, 2003, H. Nietsch
- Bachmann, Dr. med. R. M.: Natürlich gesund durch Säure-Basen-Gleichgewicht. Mit Ihrem persönlichen 7-Tage-Programm zur sanften Entsäuerung, 2001, Trias, 2. Auflage
- Bankhofer, Prof. H.: Aloe Vera: Die Pflanze für Gesundheit, Vitalität und Wohlbefinden, 2013, Kneipp-Verlag, 6. Auflage
- Barcroft, A.: Aloe Vera: Nature's Silent Healer, 2003, Baam
- Beringer, Alice: Aloe Vera – Die Königin der Heilpflanzen: Natürlich gesund und schön durch den reinen Extrakt der Aloe Vera, 2007, Heyne
- Berner, H.-G.: An vollen Töpfen verhungern, 1997, Medi Verlagsgesellschaft
- Bertram, Dr. K.: Spirulina – Die Wunderalge – Anbau, Vorkommen und Zucht, sensationelle

- Studienergebnisse, Krankheiten vorbeugen und bekämpfen, o. J., CreateSpace
- Dahlke, R.: Fasten Sie sich gesund – Das ganzheitliche Fastenprogramm, 2004, Irisana
- Dahlke, R., Ehrenberger, D.: Wege der Reinigung – Entgiften, entschlacken, loslassen, 2002, Heyne, 2. Auflage
- Delbé, J. B.: Gesund werden – gesund bleiben: Aloe-Vera-Leitfaden Gesund bleiben, 2004, M+M Verlag
- Enders, J.: Darm mit Charme, 2014, Ullstein
- **Finnegan, John &, Schmid, Rainer: Aloe Vera – das Geschenk der Natur an uns alle, 2014, Ernährung & Gesundheit, 35. Auflage**
- Frauwallner, A.: Was tun, wenn der Darm streikt? – Probiotika sinnvoll einsetzen, 2012, Kneipp-Verlag
- Gill, T.: Lieber schlank als sauer – Gesund ins Gleichgewicht mit der Säure-Basen-Diät, 2012, **CreateSpace**
- Gray, R.: Das Darmheilungsbuch – Gesundheit durch Kolon-Sanierung, 2011, Trias
- **Grillparzer, M.: Simple Detox: Das 7-Tage-Entgiftungsprogramm, 2013, Gräfe und Unzer, 5. Auflage**
- **Jester, F.: Arginin. Der natürliche Kraftstoff für Blut, Kreislauf und Gesundheit, 2010, Verlag Marina Jester**
- **Jester, F.: Chlorophyll. Das grüne Blut, Verlag Marina Jester, 2014**
- Kraske, Dr. med. E.-M.: Säure-Basen-Balance, 2008, Gräfe und Unzer, 5. Auflage
- **Liebke, Dr. F.: Doktor Chlorella! Die Alge fürs Leben. Kompendium zur Mikroalge Chlorella, Remerc & Lheiw verlagskontor, 2007**

- **Loede, P: Schlank mit Weizengras: Die Gruene-Smoothie-Weizengras-Kur, CreateSpace, 2014**
- Lohmann, M.: Der Basen-Doktor. Basische Ernährung: gezielte Hilfe bei den häufigsten Beschwerden, 2013, Trias, 2. vollst. überarb. Auflage
- **Meyer, Marianne E.: Sonnenkraft mit dem blaugrünen Lichtträger Spirulina, 2002, Windpferd, 2. Auflage**
- **Mutter, Dr. J.: Grün essen!: Die Gesundheitsrevolution auf Ihrem Teller, 2013, VAK, 3. Auflage**
- **Opitz, Ch.: Befreite Ernährung, 2013, H. Nietsch, 5. Auflage**
- **Oppermann, J.: Aloe Vera – Was die Pflanze wirklich kann, 2004, Lebensbaum**
- **Peuser, M.: Kapillaren bestimmen unser Schicksal: Aloe – Kaiserin der Heilpflanzen, Quelle für Vitalität und Gesundheit, 2010, St. Hubertus**
- **Rahn-Huber, U.: Spirulina & Chlorella: Gesund und fit mit Mikroalgen, 2015, Riwei**
- **Rahn-Huber, Ulla: Natürlich heilen und pflegen mit Aloe Vera, 2015, Riwei**
- Schneider, G. W.: Biotop Mensch – Liebe Deine Darmbakterien, 2014, Biotop Mensch, 7. Auflage
- **Simons, C. P.: Aloe Vera - 6'000 Jahre Medizingeschichte können sich nicht irren, 2015, BOD**
- **Simons, C. P.: Chlorophyll – Gesundheit ist grün, 2015, BOD**
- **Simons, C. P.: Grüner Kaffee – Garantie zum Abnehmen, 2015, BOD**
- **Simonson, B.: Gerstengrassaft: Verjüngungselixier und naturgesunder Power-Drink. Wildpferd, 15. Auflage, 2012**
- **Simonson, B.: Die Heilkraft der Afa-Alge – Vitalität für Körper und Geist, 2000, Goldmann**

- Skinner, R.: Aloe Vera: The Medicine Plant, 2005, Mill Enterprises
- Skousen, M. B.: Aloe Vera Handbook: The Acient Egyptian Medicine Plant, 2005, Book Publishing Company
- Thust, Th. M., Schlett, Dr. med. S.: Entgiften & entschlacken,
- 2006, Gräfe und Unzer
- Treutwein, N.: Übersäuerung – krank ohne Grund?, 2005, Weltbild
- Ulmer, G. A.: Gesundheitswunder Chlorophyll: Gespeicherte, gesundheitsspendende Sonnen- und Heilkraft, Ulmer, 1997
- Vollmer, J. B.: Gesunder Darm, gesundes Leben, 2010, Knaur
- Wacker, S., Wacker, Dr. med. A.: 300 Fragen zur Säure-Basen-Balance, 2013, Gräfe und Unzer, 2. Auflage
- Wagner, W.: The Chlorophyll Supplement: Alternative Medicine for a Healthy Body, 2013, Health Collection
- Wolfe, D.: Superfoods – die Medizin der Zukunft: Wie wir die machtvollsten Heiler unter den Nahrungsmitteln optimal nutzen, Goldmann, 2015

Disclaimer

Introduction

By using this book, you accept this disclaimer in full.

No advice

The book contains information. The information is not advice, and should not be treated as such.

If you think you may be suffering from any medical condition you should seek immediate medical attention. You should never delay seeking medical advice, disregard medical advice, or discontinue medical treatment because of information in the book.

No representations or warranties

To the maximum extent permitted by applicable law and subject to section below, we exclude all representations, warranties, undertakings and guarantees relating to the book.

Without prejudice to the generality of the foregoing paragraph, we do not represent, warrant, undertake or guarantee:

- that the information in the book is correct, accurate, complete or non-misleading;

- that the use of the guidance in the book will lead to any particular outcome or result.

Limitations and exclusions of liability

The limitations and exclusions of liability set out in this section and elsewhere in this disclaimer: are subject to section 6 below; and govern all liabilities arising under the disclaimer or in relation to the book, including liabilities arising in contract, in tort (including negligence) and for breach of statutory duty.

We will not be liable to you in respect of any losses arising out of any event or events beyond our reasonable control.

We will not be liable to you in respect of any business losses, including without limitation loss of or damage to profits, income, revenue, use, production, anticipated savings, business, contracts, commercial opportunities or goodwill.

We will not be liable to you in respect of any loss or corruption of any data, database or software.

We will not be liable to you in respect of any special, indirect or consequential loss or damage.

Exceptions

Nothing in this disclaimer shall: limit or exclude our liability for death or personal injury resulting from negligence; limit or exclude our liability for fraud or fraudulent misrepresentation; limit any of our liabilities in any way that is not permitted under applicable law; or exclude any of our liabilities that may not be excluded under applicable law.

Severability

If a section of this disclaimer is determined by any court or other competent authority to be unlawful and/or unenforceable, the other sections of this disclaimer continue in effect.

If any unlawful and/or unenforceable section would be lawful or enforceable if part of it were deleted, that part will be deemed to be deleted, and the rest of the section will continue in effect.

Law and jurisdiction

DISCLAIMER

This disclaimer will be governed by and construed in accordance with Swiss law, and any disputes relating to this disclaimer will be subject to the exclusive jurisdiction of the courts of Switzerland.

www.ingramcontent.com/pod-product-compliance
Lightning Source LLC
Chambersburg PA
CBHW020713180526
45163CB00008B/3062